# The
# Core Balance
# Experience

## By Harnes Stewart

# Table of Contents

# Introduction

I am Harnes Stewart, the owner of Nexxt Level Training, and I want to invite you to join me through the Core Balance Experience. Through my career as a certified personal trainer for the past twenty years, I've utilized every part of the Core Balance Technique to achieve in the area of fitness as well as in other areas of my life. My hope in writing this book is to show that the Core Balance Experience is more than just a technique to train by, it is a life experience. I have spent considerable time developing this powerful concept, to ensure my clients not only improve their fitness, but also gain knowledge and whole-life balance with it.

In this book, I will walk you through every step of the system. The first part we will embark upon together is what the Core Balance

Experience is. Here, you will get a basic understanding of the technical aspects of Core Balance—the technique, balance, posture, and areas of focus—as well as the value of the journey, what it brings into your life, and how the results elevate you physically and mentally, to make you a better person.

The second part focuses on how the Core Balance Technique and Experience differ from any other technique. I don't say that to invalidate the value of other techniques, because I believe other products work and have purpose too. However, the Core Balance Technique is different in many ways.

The first difference I love is how it allows you to familiarize your body with different exercises and things that will work for you in achieving your personal goals. Not everything will work for you, but this technique will enable you to find what will work for your body and what will best help your body change.

Second, the Core Balance Experience focuses on the positive and negative ranges. I'm going to teach you how using negative and positive work within the same realm in your workout doubles the effect of doing reps no matter what the exercise is. This means you can get increased results—half the effort and double the reward.

Third, I want to show you how CBE is different in allowing you to protect your lower back. The lower back is a valuable part of your body because it holds so much weight, requiring balance in that area. This technique shows you how to balance by using your abdominal region, proper posture, and knee balance.

This allows you not only to protect your lower back, but also to help you balance out what you're doing with your core. These differences give us an advantage in reaching our goals.

The next several sections will focus on how the CBE works to improve your overall life experiences. It is broken down into three separate sections: the mind, the body, and the spirit. The first portion is about the mental benefits of Core Balance. I'll show you that the Core Balance Experience takes a different mental approach. We will learn how this type of technique affects your mind, which elevates you to another place mentally to be able to look at fitness differently. You will not only be able to look at life differently, but also to let your fitness experience become a life experience within you. I will show you how to build a new mindset, one that allows you to move forward in every area of your life, no matter what you face. If we can change the way you think about overall fitness and well-being, we can help you accomplish things you once thought impossible.

The second part is a focus on the body, the physical benefits of training with the CBE. This doesn't just pertain to the visual result, the body transformation people want to see from their hard work. It is also about the general health aspects. Developing Core Balance enhances flexibility, strength, and endurance. Realistically, not every male is going to have a big muscular transformation, and every female will not become a fashion model. Each person has different dynamics. I believe in these techniques because they produce balance from the center, both physically and mentally. Understanding this will help you identify your goals and gather physicality and will give your journey a greater purpose.

The third segment is about the spirit. We will explore how you can connect mind, body, and spirit for overall health and wellness. I believe true health is found when you are spiritually healthy in addition to being physically and mentally fit. In fact, I believe the spiritual aspect is what will ultimately take you to the next level. I just want you to know that from a faith standpoint, I'm a faithful believer in Jesus Christ. I believe that when you connect your God-given purpose to your health and fitness goals, God will not only help you develop the mental and the physical aspects, but will also propel you spiritually and take you to a place where all three aspects work together. When you combine mental, physical, and spiritual strength, you become a powerful person. My goal is to assist you in doing that!

The CBE is a six-week system comprised of six major workouts that build from your core strength. I built the system based on my personal experiences in the gym over the past twenty years. Each week's workout is designed to establish a foundational stage you can build upon the following week. It is systematically calculated to push you to the next level.

The first workout in my system is called the *measuring stick*. With it, we start measuring your abilities—finding your strengths and which exercises work best for your body. Weeks two through five will build on those strengths, add flexibility and lean muscle, increase your endurance, and test your limits. The final workout of the six weeks is a workout simply called *weight*. In this workout we increase the weights in order to evaluate and test the resistance in the foundation you have built over the first five weeks. I believe this system offers what you need to transform your life, health, and fitness goals. At forty-six years of age, I am in the best shape ever. This system can diversify into different things, like a chameleon. It is very beautiful, but it requires a complete effort of the total system. I use it daily in my workouts, and to transform the people I physically train so they meet the goals they personally set at their initial evaluation with me.

Our final discussion will focus on the actual benefits, or the fruits, produced at the back end of your journey through the Core Balance Experience. I'll talk about how to make your workout cleaner and shorter, how to be more efficient within your workout, and finally, how to manage your space. There is nothing like becoming the ultimate manager over not only your fitness goals but also the other areas of your life.

I call this system the Core Balance Experience because it is meant to bring you structure and the ability to gain knowledge in finding your greater purpose. It will connect your purpose and goals with something greater than yourself. When you get the spirit, body, and mind working in conjunction with one another, you will inevitably become a better human being. This is the whole reason we put this product together. I believe the CBE is a powerful product that will help change the way you look at health and fitness. I feel it will take you to the next level of fitness as well as any other area of your life. So let's get started!

# What Is the Core Balance Technique?

Core Balance Training is an art form of technique and movement in fitness. It's learning how to work through a technique or a circuit for optimal results. Throughout this book I will break it down for you based on my twenty years of experience of using the Core Balance Technique. Right now, at the age of forty-six, I think I am in the best shape of my life. The things I have learned from Core Balance and this technique have really accelerated my fitness experience and have made me stable and structurally strong.

## Technical Aspects of the Core Balance Experience and Technique

When we talk about the *core*, we are usually talking about the midsection of your body: the abdominals *and* the lower back region. I believe Core Balance is the ability to engage your abdominal region simultaneously with your lower back in various exercises to help balance out those movements. (See figs. 1 and 2 on the following pages for improper and proper Core Balance.)

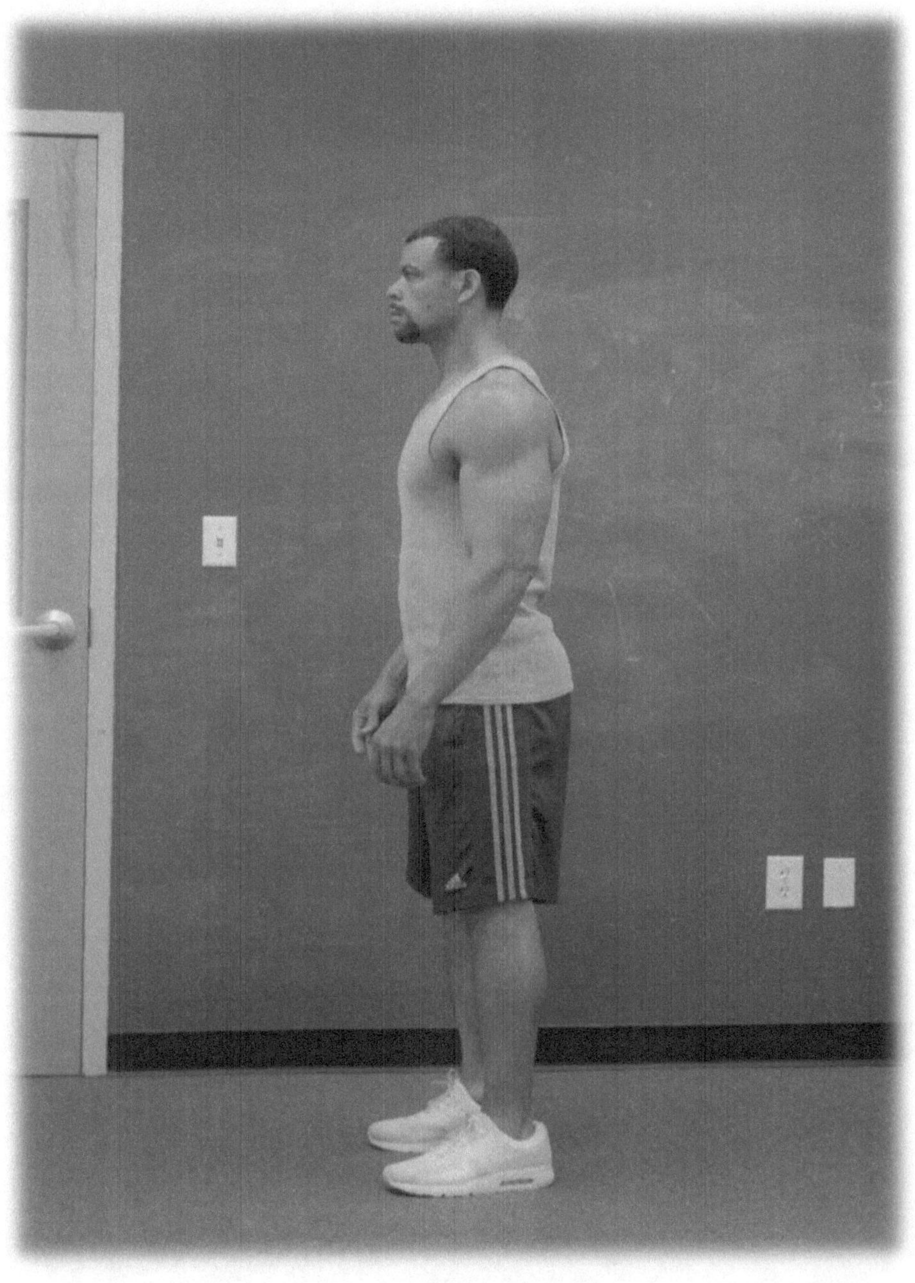

*Figure 1:  Improper Core Balance*

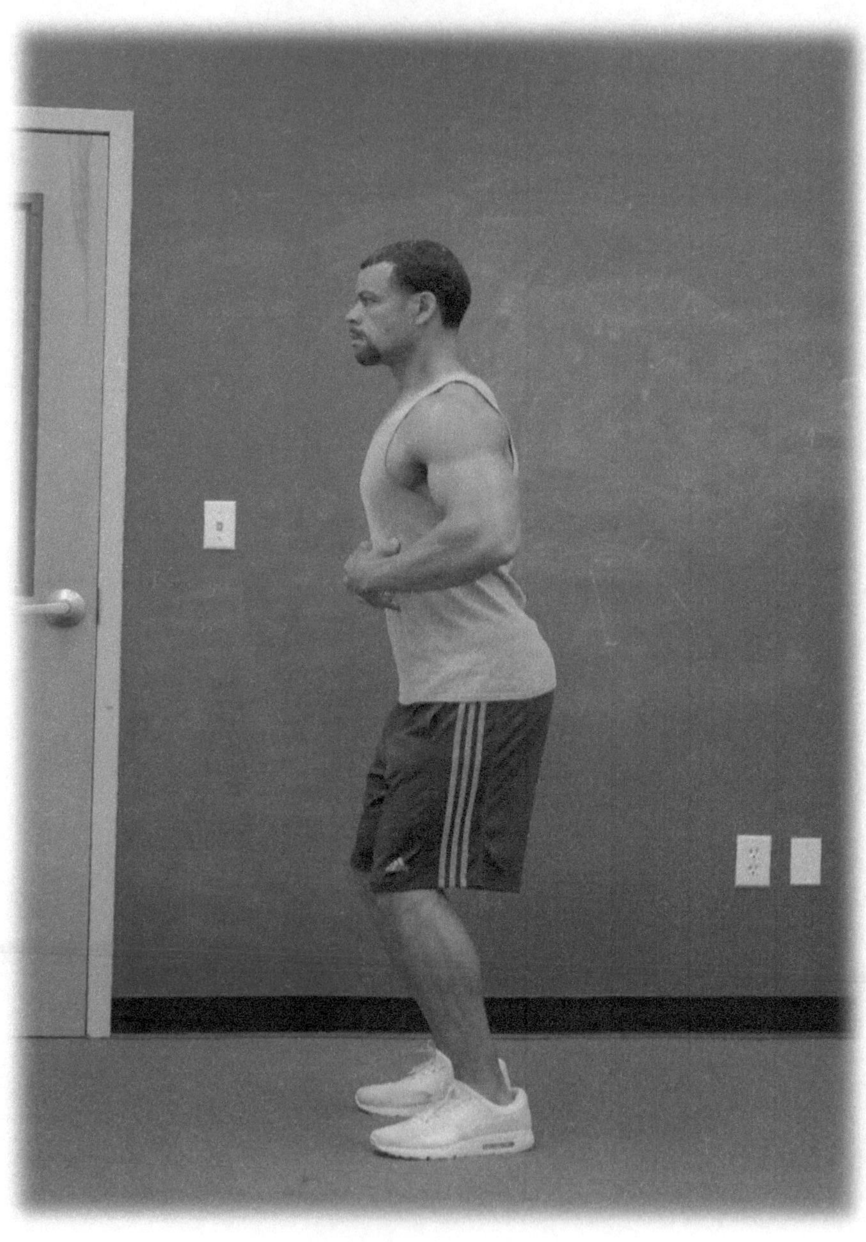

*Figure 1: Proper Core Balance*

You can see from the pictures that Core Balance is based on having an upright core when you do certain exercises and having something called *knee balance*. This means your knees are not straight when you lift, but instead, you will use a little bit of knee balance to protect your lower back and also engage your core. It increases your posture to the point that when you do exercises using the correct Core Balance, you maximize the potential of those exercises. I teach something I believe is not very traditional from a Core Balance standpoint: you have to engage your core, be upright, and bend your knees slightly, to avoid damaging your lower back. Bending your knees a little bit allows your legs to absorb any extra weight or pressure instead of your lower back.

Core Balance allows you to have both technique and balance. Your exercises will occur between your shoulders instead of outside of them. Core Balance allows you to do all the exercises in front of your body. I say this because many things we do as human beings are done right in front of us. Just think about it: driving, putting on makeup, and cooking are all activities that exist within the range of our shoulders.

When it comes down to lifting and using the technique, I do not believe in the wide-leg approach. I believe in an approach where your feet are lined up with your shoulders, in a relaxed position and using some knee balance (fig. 3 and 4).

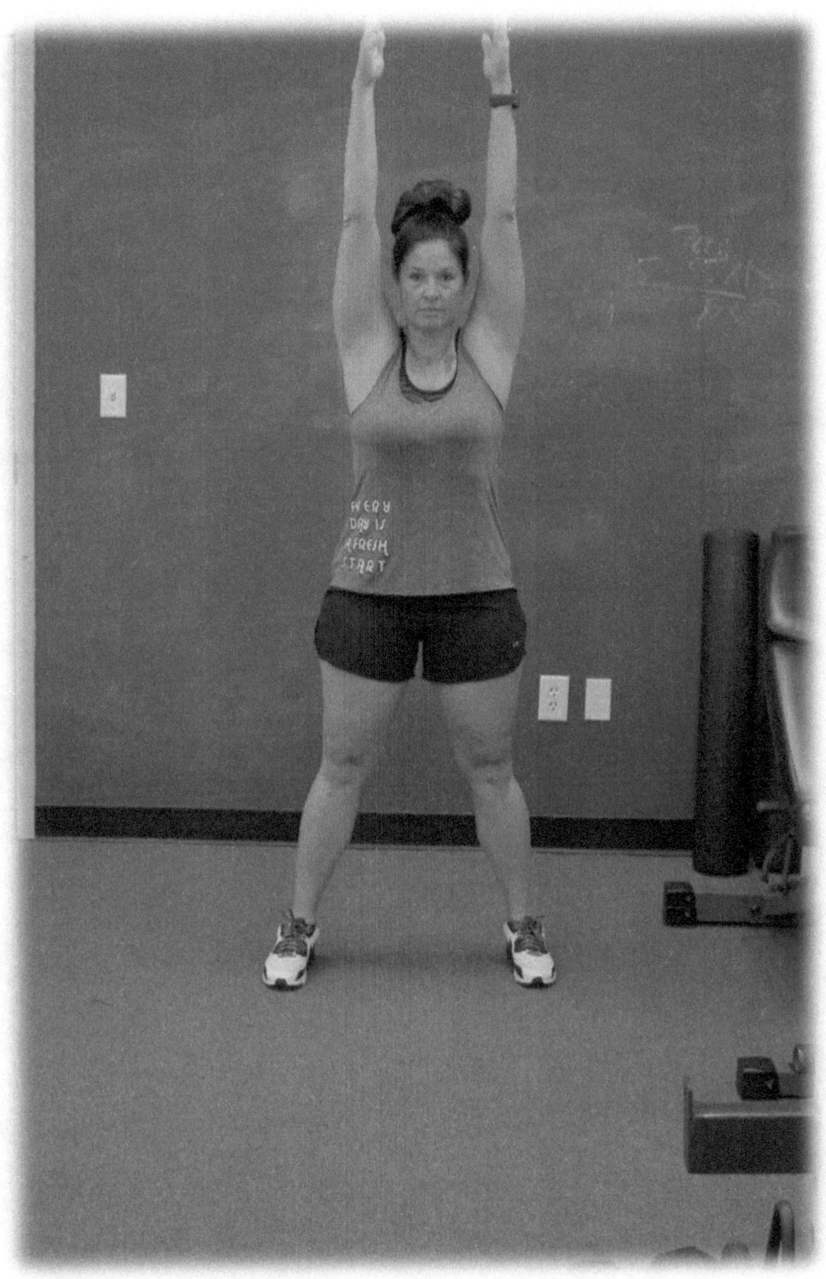

*Figure 3: Wide leg approach*

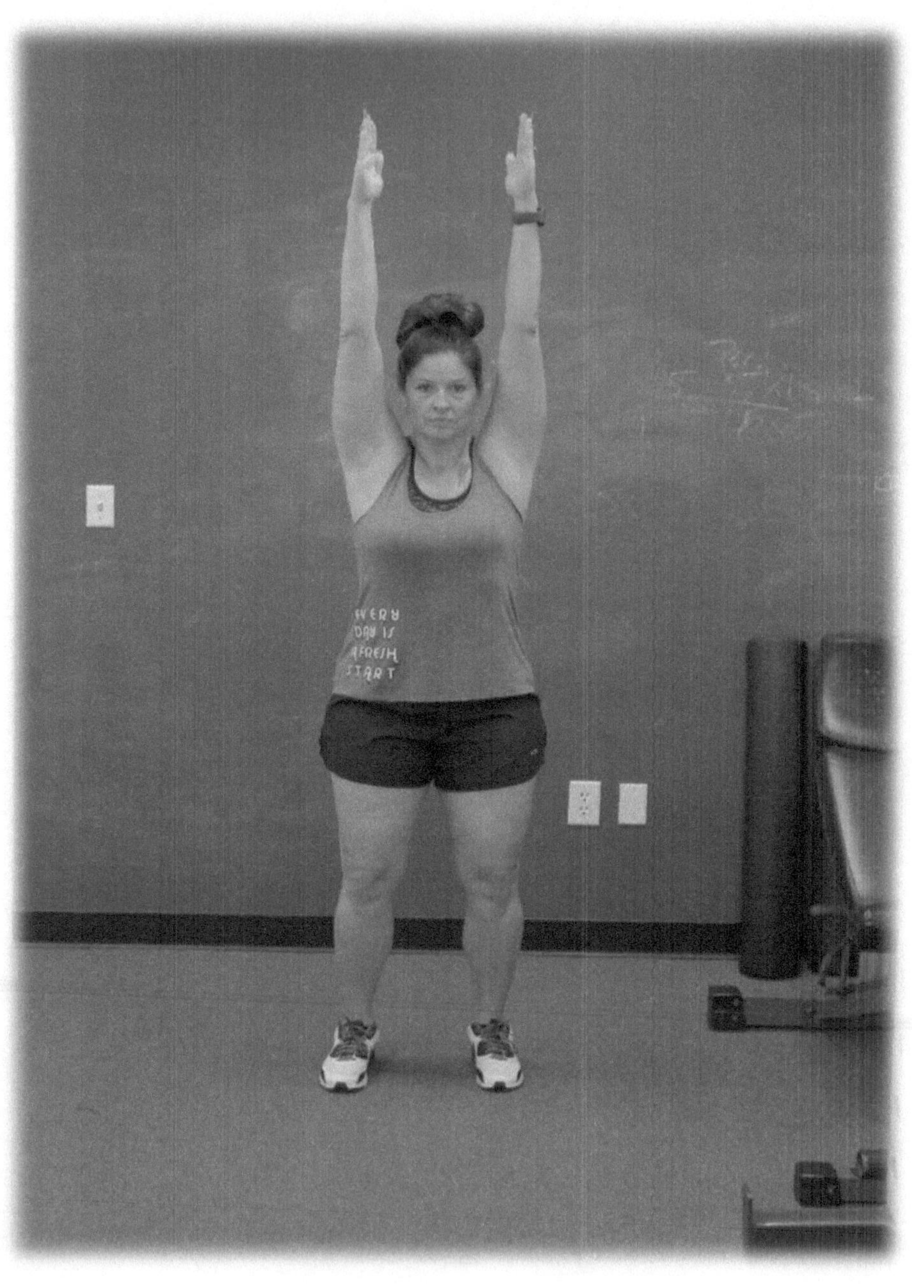


*Figure 4: Core Balance Approach*

This allows you to have perfect range in different exercises, where everything is right in front of you. I have learned that by keeping everything in the center when you do these exercises, you are also working your abs. As you begin to understand what this technique really is, it will revolutionize the way you build lean muscle. You will be able to grow lean muscle at a rate you have never been able to before. Now that I understand this, many of my exercises are not based on resistance, but rather on technique and leverage.

The Core Technique gives me leverage over all the different exercises I do. It allows me to bring more value to the equipment than the equipment brings to me. I want you to realize the Core Technique is not about resistance. Rather, it is all about you bringing value to the equipment by using a technique that will help you get to a certain point. Once you reach that certain point, you can get to the next level. The actual technique makes sense when you are able to get involved with your core and do a volume of different exercises from a technical standpoint.

When you start using Core Balance and maintaining an upright core, you get to a point where you can dominate the exercises you do. You will go into your workout with confidence and understanding. Even if you just pick up a couple of dumbbells, the technique will give you more value in all of your exercises.

There are two reasons why it is good to stay in your shoulder range, as follows:

1. Flow - When you have the confidence that you can keep this range, you can flow easily through the exercises.

2. It protects you from injury. That is a crucial part of the Core Balance Technique, because many of the injuries in the gym are shoulder injuries.

This is because we lift so far from the center of our bodies that we injure our shoulders. Almost all of the chest and shoulder injuries occur because we lift out of our shoulder range.

In my twenty years of experience, I can tell you that the Core Balance Technique will revolutionize you and will take you to another level in fitness and training where you have never been before.

## The Journey: Learning about Your Body

The second part I want to talk about is the journey. The journey is learning about your own body. You will learn what exercise and what pieces of equipment work to accelerate what you are looking for in regard to your goals.

When I bring somebody in, I teach them how to do pushups within the range of their shoulders rather than out. I teach them how to get the core involved and how to find the range their bodies allow them to have. Then we begin to build confidence, and the range and strength will increase. Soon they find out that everything can be and will be facilitated through their core and through their balance.

I may not know what your specific goals are, but regardless of your fitness level, you will find exercises that work for **your** body. This is like when you go into a shoe store and see many shoes in different colors, sizes, and shapes. You may see many you like, but not all of them will fit the way you want them to.

The same goes for exercise and fitness: there are lots of exercises and ways to exercise, but not everything will be for you. However, when you use the Core Balance Technique, you will be capable of maximizing **any** exercise you do. It does not matter if you are a beginner or an expert.

People from all levels can benefit from using the Core Balance Technique.

I really get excited to teach this technique to my clients, because once I do, they begin a journey. This takes the mental weight off of you. It doesn't matter if you don't know what to do; you can learn what exercises work for you and what exercises do not. It's okay if an exercise isn't for you, because not everything will work for everyone. Remember, in the same way we are all different, your exercises can be different too. It's okay when you have to leave an exercise that does not fit with your range or your balance.

Once you reach this point, you can do a circuit based on your core and balance to create a workout experience that has great value to *your* body. You will leave the gym so confident, that you can learn outside of the box. Many times people plateau because they are inside a box. They are stuck in standard techniques and cannot find what exercises work for them. What is beautiful about the Core Balance Technique is that it will allow you to diversify and find many different exercises that will work for you, whether that is ropes, the bar, or dumbbells. Whatever your favorite is, it will work because you are not founding yourself in the equipment. Instead, your foundation is in your technique. This will maximize your exercises and will get you to the desired results of your goal.

I find this very exciting, and once you start to see the results, I think you will too. Now that you understand more about what Core Balance actually is, let's talk about how it differs from other techniques.

# How the Core Balance Technique Differs from Other Techniques

In this section, I want to talk about how Core Balance training is different from other techniques. I am not saying other techniques do not work. However, the Core Balance Experience has given me the ability to consistently achieve my fitness goals. It has also allowed me to clarify and accelerate at a pace many other techniques haven't. Because of this, I teach it exclusively.

When we talk about the Core Balance Technique, we refer to the engagement of your core when you do certain things. This means being in an upright position with your abs and applying something called *knee balance*. When I say *knee balance*, I mean avoiding positions where your knees are locked when doing any type of workout or lifting. You should avoid locking your knees, because doing so puts a lot of pressure on your lower back. I have found over the years that it is important not only to use the correct core technique, but also to use knee balance. Both of these things can absorb some of the pressure on your lower back, balancing everything.

Now let's get into how Core Balance is different from other workouts.

1. **What Core Balance has done for me over the years and what it will do for you.**

Core Balance will show you how to familiarize your body with movements. Many times when you are lifting weights or when you are doing exercises, you don't have the correct range. That range in movement is important. I was missing a lot of range in my early days, because my technique was terrible. However, when I learned the Core Balance Technique, I gained the ability to familiarize my body with the correct movements, no matter the exercise.

Let me give you an example. If I am using dumbbells to do a chest press or bench press, I must involve my core in order to achieve proper range. Involving my core naturally elevates my chest because my shoulders are slightly back, and this forces the weights to rest about an inch above my chest when my arms are down at a ninety-degree angle. This allows the lift to be pushed up and through rather than being forced out and around in a form that is too wide to achieve maximum range. I found this provided me with an additional two and a half to three inches of range in my lift that enabled me to develop lean muscle much more quickly. (See figs. 5 and 6 for proper and improper dumbbell technique.)

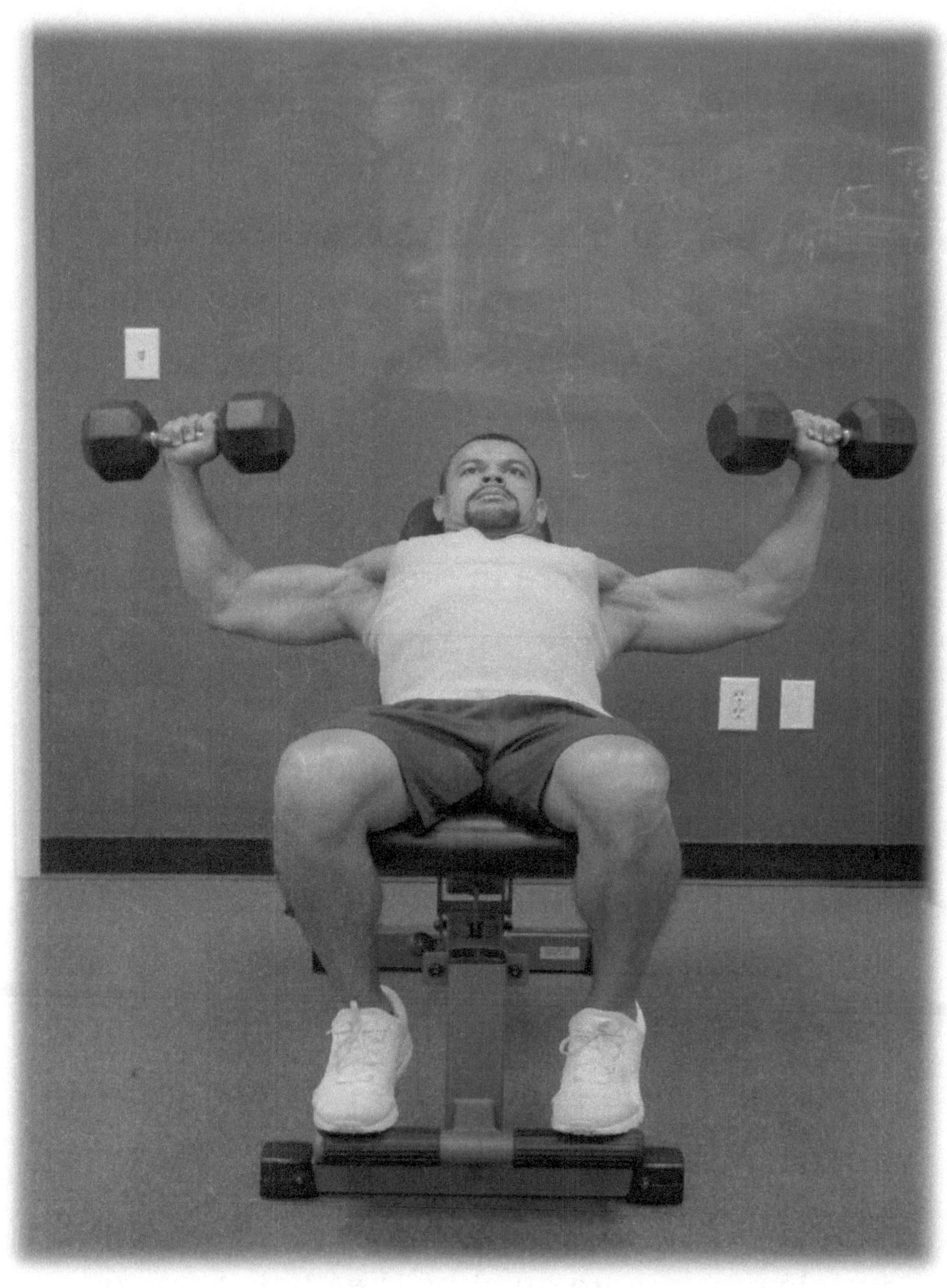

*Figure 5: Improper Dumbbell Press Technique*

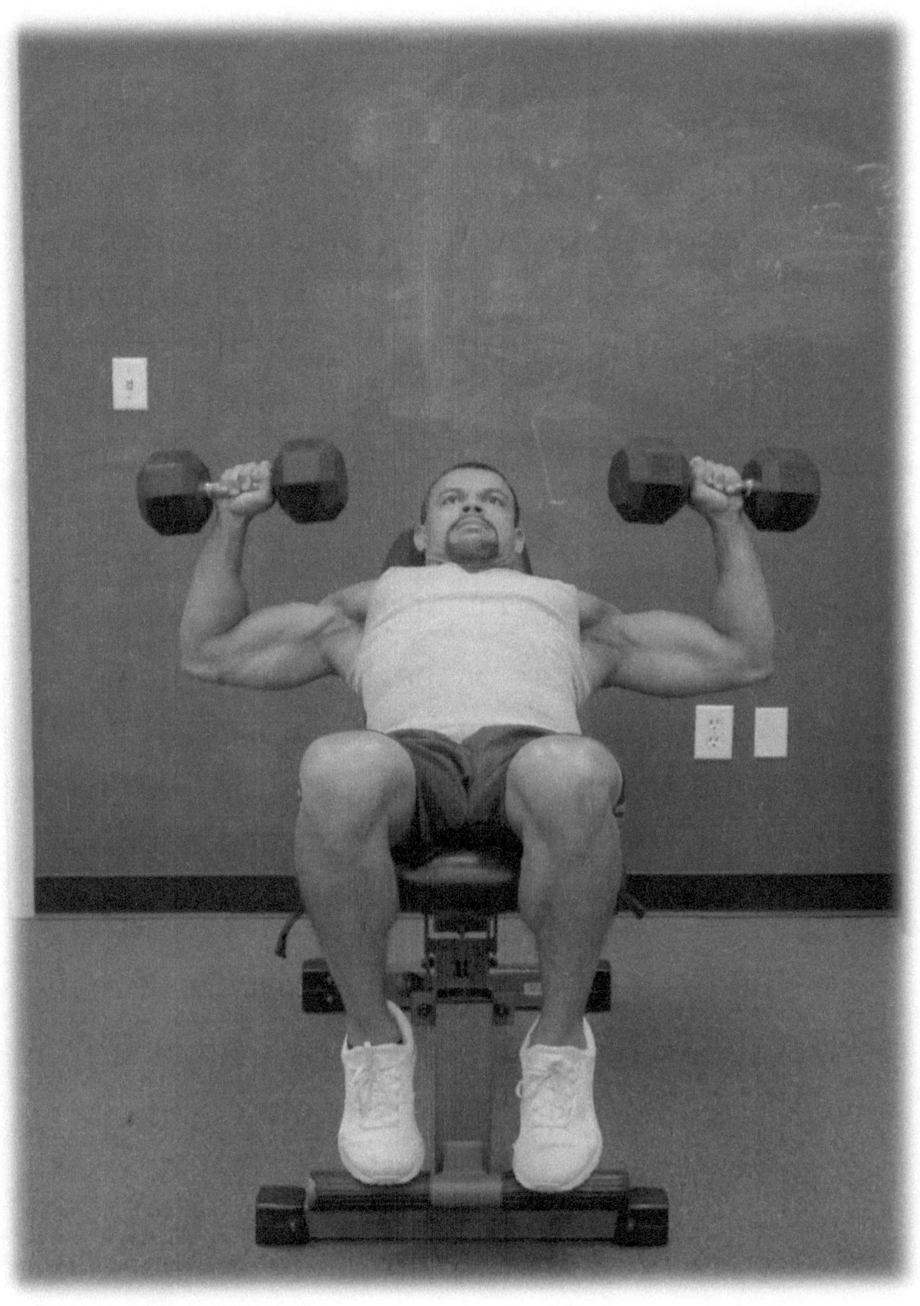

*Figure 6: Core Balance Dumbbell Press Technique*

When you familiarize yourself with the proper form, technique, and balance, it will become second nature to you. It becomes as simple as putting on your clothes. You will remember the movements and aspects of each lift through proper technique, which enables you to utilize appropriate form when transferring weight in an everyday lift, like picking up a child or a heavy box. Picking up weight causes your base, abdominal region, and back to bear the resistance or "carry the burden" of that weight. One of two things will happen with this resistance: you will either stand still in a postured position with Core Balance, or you will be off center and your body will tilt because you are off balance.

If you tilt it means that your base can't really sustain the weight you have. If you stand still, it lets you know your core is strong enough to handle that weight.

Why am I telling you this? When you use the Core Balance Technique, you keep everything centered in your shoulders, and your body is upright with knee balance. This allows everything to stay in front of you. Even if it is on top of you and you are laying some resistance down, it allows the weight to balance through your core and through you lower back. It's a powerful technique, and over my years of doing different workouts, I have been able to figure out the correct range for different exercises and the art of getting something from point A to point B. I think that has absolutely revolutionized everything I've done.

The number one thing this has done for me is allowed me to grow the muscles and areas I wanted to grow without having to lift as much weight. This technique taught me I did not need to put X amount of weight to get X amount of big or strong or flexible or to burn X amount of calories. It really took the shackles off me in terms of what I could do with my level of fitness.

It has also allowed me to walk through workouts with confidence. When you know that as long as you have the right range, you're maximizing what you have and learning the different aspects of it, everything will be easier for you. Today, at the age of forty-six, I am still able to do things I did when I was twenty. I might not lift the same weight, but I know I can do it correctly, and my body still sustains the lean muscle, balance, and technique to continue working out at a high level. I can do this because my body is familiar with the lifts.

I know you go to the gym and all these machines look like they do the same thing. However, when you learn the technique and you learn the machines, you learn the range of them. When you learn how to use a machine and find a way that it works for your body, you will never have a problem as far as achieving your goals, no matter what they are from a fitness standpoint.

2. **It allows you to put together positive and negative range.**

The second difference is the ability to use a positive and negative range together. If you don't know what that means, I'll explain. When you do a lift, there is a positive part when you push the weight off you, and there's also the negative aspect when you bring the weight down to you. Whether it's pulling something to you or letting something pull you back to it, there is a positive and a negative flow. When you use the Core Balance Technique and you have proper knee balance, which I call *sprinter's balance*, and when you're engaging your core and allowing any type of resistance to come to you, you are getting the negative when it comes down plus positive when you push out. That is important because now you are getting double the value of the lift in any type of exercise you may use to achieve your goals. By leveraging your lifts this way, you'll find it does not take that much weight to achieve the result you want, even though it looks like it does. (See figs. 7 and 8 for positive and negative range.)

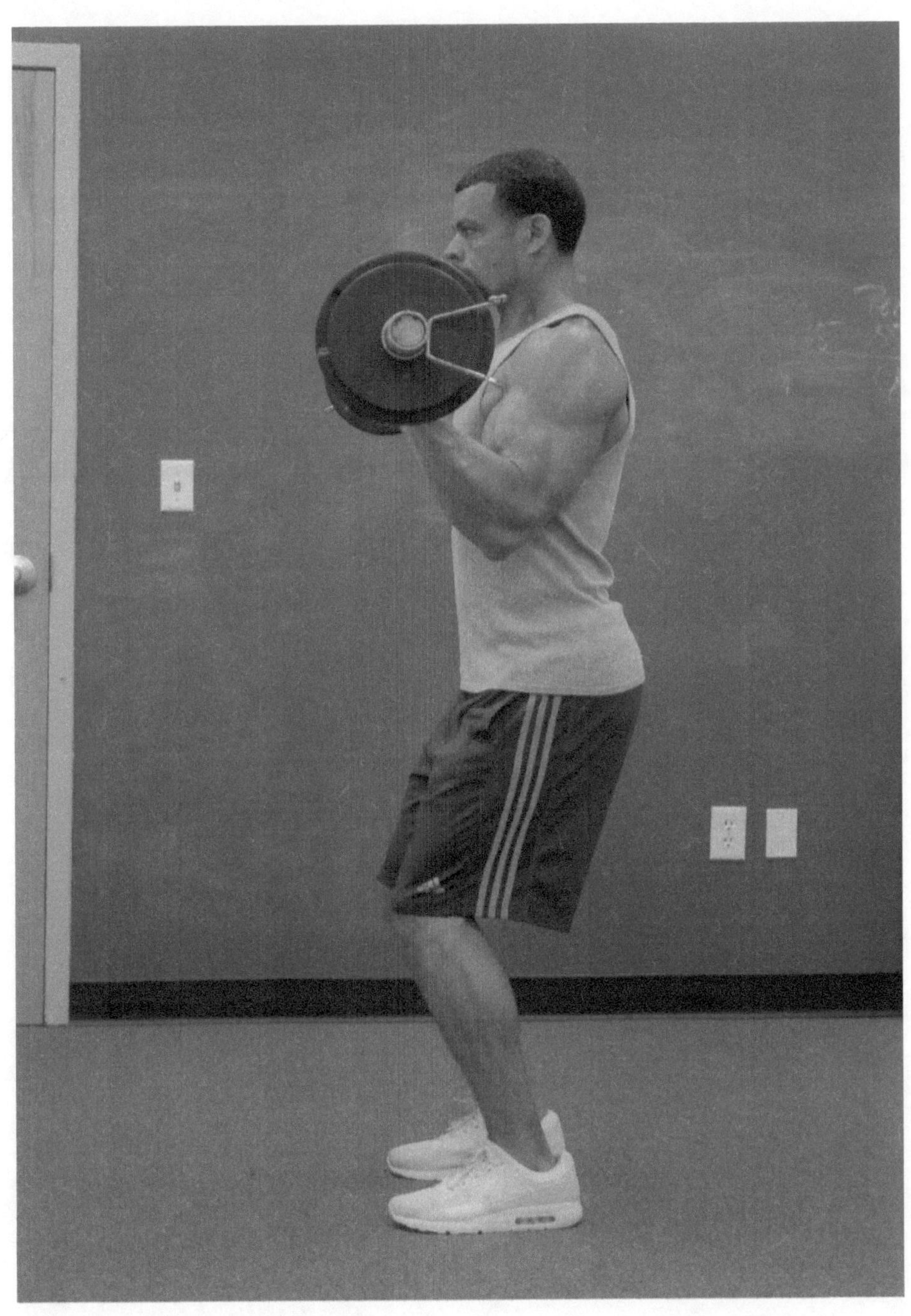

*Figure 7: Positive Range*

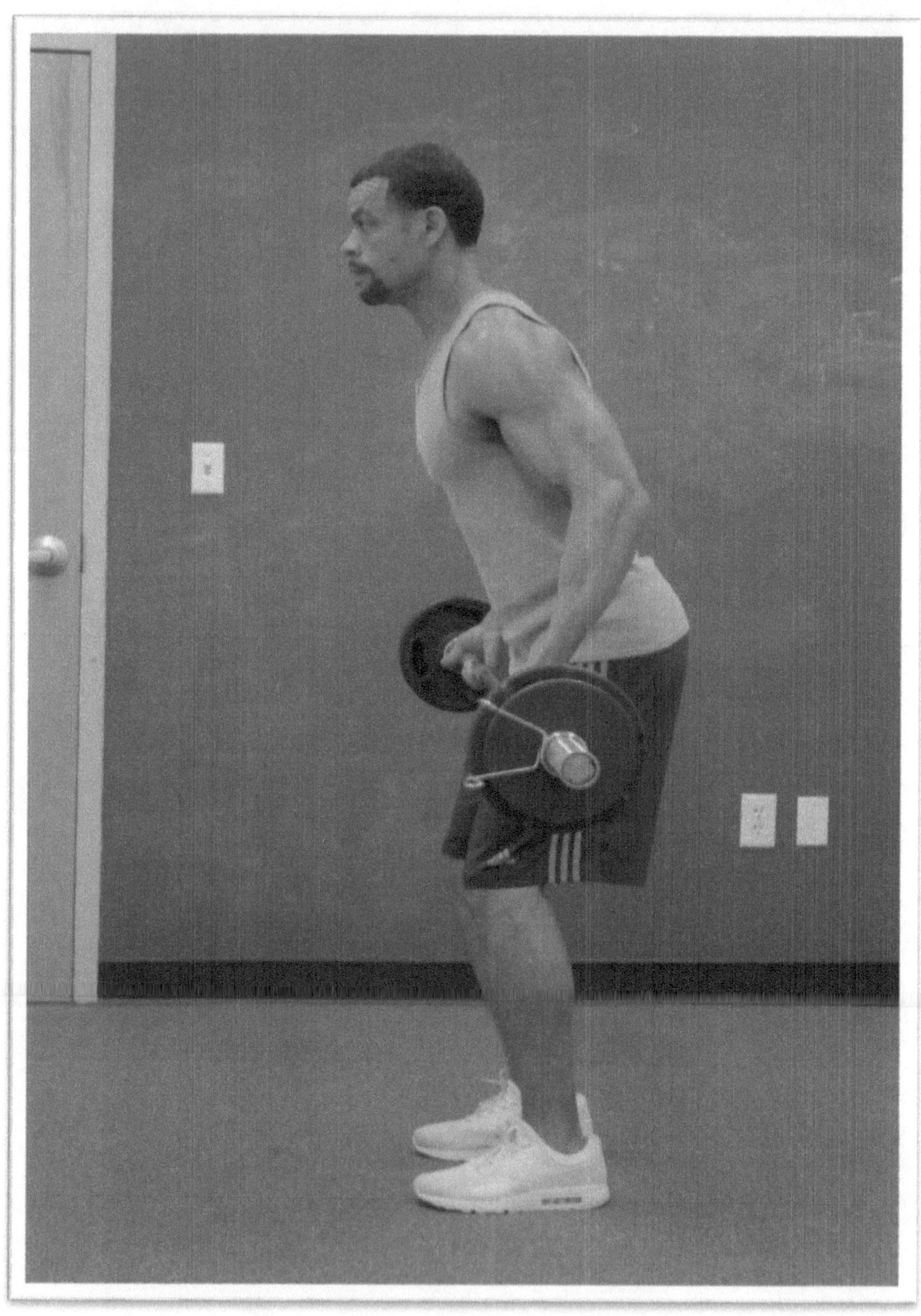

*Figure 8:  Negative Range*

When you can maximize what it looks like to do a lift and you can control the positive and negative in it, you have double the value of what you are doing. You can turn a set of ten into a set of twenty because now you are definitely getting double the value from the positive and negative range. I call it getting from A to B.

When you master the art of the exercise with control, both positive and negative, you will see results 50 percent faster than with some of the traditional techniques. This is what's special about the Core Balance Technique. The mindset of it lets you understand that you don't have to be scared to go to a piece of equipment and learn how to use it, and you also don't have to go so fast or so slow. You are looking for the controlled movement and what that does every time you do an exercise. You can utilize both the positive and negative range and get the maximum value of both with this technique.

### 3. **It protects your lower back.**

The third difference is the Core Balance Technique protects your lower back. This is the most critical aspect of these points because the lower back is one of the most important parts of the body in regard to fitness. Protecting your lower back comes from having correct posture. Proper Core Balance posture is when you are standing with your head and chest up, knees slightly bent, and both feet aligned with your shoulders. This is not a wide stance, but one where your legs and feet create an invisible line from your shoulders down to the floor. The Core Balance Technique focuses on positioning your body in a manner that releases the pressure from your lower back, which in turn provides the abdominal region with the ability to assist with balance, control, and support. When your core is tight and working with the lower back, you can bend without causing injury.

Think about it. Have you ever woken up one morning with a pulled muscle in your neck or back? It is unlikely the product of a sudden movement in your sleep; rather, it usually stems from lying in a position with poor posture. An extended period of compromised posture forces unusual pressure on the muscles, which results in a strain—extreme tightness that prohibits your natural movements. If you have a pulled muscle in your lower back, it affects your body's movement in terms of walking, sitting, standing, and bending. The same is true with lifting weights. If you are leaning too far over or standing with an overly wide stance when lifting weights, the repetition of lifting from a compromised position will produce strained lower back muscles. Practicing the proper Core Balance stance will protect your lower back when you bend down, both in the fitness arena and in your daily activities. When your core is tight and working with the lower back, it enables you to bend without injury.

Additionally, proper technique is necessary for supporting resistance over your head. It creates a solid base and the perfect alignment that stabilizes the body for doing a variety of exercises and lifts. The Core Technique facilitates the abdominal region's ability to work in conjunction with the lower back as a cohesive unit. This foundational stance puts any person in control of the lift. This control is found in the range of the lift, and anyone can find it at any level of training. I believe that if you use this technique, whether you are bending down to do a squat or bending over to pick up something on the floor, it will protect your lower back from injury.

# The Mental Benefits of the Core Balance Technique

This is going to be a powerful section. If you grab this, you are really going to get what is going on. I own a company called Nexxt Level Training, and we build three aspects: mind, body, and spirit. Once you have the conjunction of these three working together, you can accomplish anything you want in any aspect of your life.

When we start talking about the Core Balance Experience, we refer to more than just a technique. We call it an *experience* because it takes you to another level in your life. There are four main mental benefits the Core Balance Experience will contribute to your life, which we will discuss in detail now.

## 1. **Discipline**

I want to talk to you about how the Core Balance Experience affects the mind. It affects it in a positive way that moves you or accelerates you toward your goals. Because this technique creates balance between your core and your lower back, and knee balance to help the flow through exercises, the number one thing it does is creates something called *discipline*.

Once you learn the art of this technique, it begins to work for you in your workouts. You can see how many calories you can burn and how your heart can accelerate at different levels and be really efficient in all of those levels, while getting a multitude of different things done.

This gives you the discipline to think about your exercises rather than how difficult your exercises are every time you get ready to work out. Your concern will be how you are going to get Core Balance established before you get into each exercise, and then you are going to dominate each exercise with your balance and range. All of this comes from having the proper Core Balance Technique.

But it doesn't stop there. What I have learned over the years is that investing in this program has not only given me discipline in the gym, but in other areas of my life as well. Every day when I go to the gym, I focus on a workout and on my core. This focus and discipline creates a balance that follows me even outside the gym. I also think about the balance of things. When you get the balance of things, you are not easily influenced. That means you can't be swayed too much to the right or to the left.

Now, I realize you are only human. Sometimes you won't want to work out every day, and some days you're going to feel that you can go more than other days. Other days your system will not feel like it usually does, or your nutrition will be off and you won't feel as energetic as usual. But in general, when you get this system down, you will create discipline, which will give you balance. You will be as disciplined as you want to be. When you go to the gym or to work out or anywhere else, you will look at everything from the center.

The mental aspect is something Core Balance works on. I see this with my clients all the time. We always work with the mind, putting something positive in there, and will always use the core. I accelerate the environment by approaching my clients with the maximum amount of energy so they can find the maximum amount of range, either negative or positive. We do this so people can get to the point where everything becomes so disciplined they always feel like they can dominate when trying to reach their goals.

## 2. **It creates commitment.**

If you begin Core Balance Training, you will be 100 percent committed because once you start seeing the proof and the results of this training, you will be fully on board with it.

You will walk into the gym with a mindset that will facilitate every exercise you do, regardless of the part of the body you are working on. This is true even if your exercises are very diverse and you do different exercises every time.

The beauty of this type of training is that it also facilitates your commitment toward other things, like your relationships and other things that are valuable to you, as well as the things you want to accomplish in a day. This training has allowed me to look at things differently. Now I don't give up easily when I stand up to obstacles;

instead, I *commit* to them. This technique allows you to endure. When you can enjoy and learn the value of what works for your body, your commitment goes to another level.

## 3. **It creates *oneness*.**

Everyone has goals. They are not necessarily fitness goals, but they are goals, something someone really wants to achieve. When it comes down to fitness, there are many types of goals. Not everyone wants to lose weight; some want to get lean. Some people want to gain weight, some people want balance, some people want posture, and some just want the ability to have proportionate muscle and lean muscle working at the same time.

The reason I teach people Core Balance is because it takes their goals and this technique and brings them into oneness. When you get these two working together, you have someone in a position where they can get to the next level. The oneness creates the path, and when you get a committed person who learns the art of Core Balance, they are going to find the oneness of what it takes to reach their goals.

When you reach this point, it is exciting. And when you get excited and you get what I'm trying to tell you, it creates a mindset. No matter where you are trying to get in life, if you take your goal and the technique I will teach you, you can put them together with a commitment to follow through and achieve what you want.

## 4. **It gives you diversity.**

I often run into clients that tell me, "I've been lifting for so and so time and I've reached a plateau. I really can't lose any more weight, get any more lean muscle, or gain any more flexibility." I understand they are talking about *plateauing*. That happens when you keep doing the traditional workouts and you can't reach a higher level of fitness or get out of your box. It is like eating the same food every single day. If you eat pizza or broccoli every day, after a while it gets a little bit boring and you want to know how to be more creative.

Plateaus are not a problem with Core Balance because of the diversity it allows for. This is one of the main reasons I'm so glad I learned this technique. It allows you to be versatile. One week you can do it one way, but the next week you can do it another way. The Core Balance Technique facilitates the use of many different exercises, and you can recombine certain exercises to work on different areas of your body. All of these will work for you in many different ways. Your exercises aren't dominated by the machines, but instead are dominated by your core.

One of the benefits of Core Balance Training is that it creates a mindset for you to move forward in discipline. It allows you to become committed, to come into a oneness with your purpose and your goal, and to diversify. That means you can get very creative with the way you do exercises. Because you are doing them from your core, your balance gives you complete protection. It also gives your mind the ability to understand that you can go to the next level.

Now that you know the mental benefits to the Core Balance Experience, let's move on to the physical benefits.

# The Physical Benefits of the Core Balance Technique

This second benefit of the Core Experience that I want to talk about is how it benefits your body physically. These are the benefits most people will be interested in when talking about a workout, since most of your goals are around losing weight, getting stronger, gaining flexibility, etc. If you have a certain fitness goal, you want to see the actual fruit or tangible evidence of the work you put into reaching it, so the physical benefit is important.

In terms of the Core Balance Experience, there are six main ways you will benefit physically, which I will break down for you below:

# 1. Posture

The first thing I want to break down is the posture. As a trainer, I often run into people that have terrible posture. This is mostly because of their jobs or due to bad habits. Anyone can fall into this category. One thing the Core Balance Technique teaches your body is how to have *perfect posture*. This is due to the knee balance and the engagement of the core and doing exercises where you are upright. When you have this type of posture, it allows you to be upright and strong in your presentation when you meet people. It also gives you leverage when you are doing exercises.

I want to focus in this area because posture is very important to the Core Balance Technique. In the gym, if you have bad posture, whether you do chest, triceps, or legs, it could greatly impact whether you get the value of the complete range of your exercises. There were many times in my past that I didn't get anything out of a workout because of my bad posture. It took me a long time to learn what I was doing wrong. Luckily for you, you are already one step ahead by using this program.

One of the things I teach is having proper posture within the range of what you're doing in your lift. That is a powerful aspect of what we do with the Core Balance Technique.

## 2. Strength

Second, I want to point out strength. Many people look for strength in every area of their bodies. Many people can notice that after two or three weeks of training they are stronger than when they started. That gets people very excited. When people see that they are getting stronger and bigger, it will keep them going. They become confident, and it pushes them to the next level.

When you are operating with a technique that allows your core to direct the flow of getting energy out, all of your energy is then centralized within the confines of your shoulders. There is more power flowing from the range found when you are working from proper core-balanced posture (closer to the body) versus a wider stance. This technique centralizes that strength and adds power to any lift you may do because you are working from your core. That Core Balance combines all your strength within the proper area of range, so you can actually find a place that builds and transforms your body. I teach this technique in every exercise because it produces results. Be assured, this technique strengthens you. When you can manifest your strength, you benefit by being able to build your entire body faster.

When your energy is centered, going through your core, and your posture is great, you don't have to worry about your energy flow that's out of your reach. You only have to worry about the energy in the area closer to you because it flows equally.

That is why this technique is really so powerful.

## 3. Building Proportional Lean Muscle

When I talk about building *proportional lean muscle*, I am not just talking about building lean muscle. You often see people whose upper body is big but their lower body is skinny, or their lower body is big and their upper body skinny. These people have centralized great effort into an area of fitness, but are lacking in other areas.

The Core Balance Technique allows you to flow from your core and demands upright posture. It increases your ability to build your shoulders, back, chest, and legs. I'm not just talking about building just to get big; I am also talking about a woman building lean muscle structure, with proportion. What this does is create balance, so your body will grow in balance. That means you will get as much in the right as you will get in the left; the proportion of the right side will be equal to the left side. When you use this technique, it allows you to be balanced. Every exercise will work for you.

I personally work out five times a week, doing very short fifty-minute workouts. Using this technique allows me to do every part of my body very proportionally, building every area, so one part is not bigger than the other.

As you balance out what you are doing and you allow yourself to learn the art of this technique, you will see over a period of time that your muscles will build very proportionally.

## 4. Flexibility

Flexibility, or a person's range of motion, is extremely important when exercising. When I say *range of motion*, I mean their ability to move freely in both their muscles and joints. From my experience, it is often not until people begin their fitness journey that they realize how much of their flexibility has been lost. They are unable to bend or stretch because over an extended period of time, the lack of intentionally focusing on these movements has caused the muscles and joints to become restricted and less limber. They are collectively unable to function at a full range of motion. When flexibility is lost, the body is more at risk of injury. The Core Balance Technique works to stretch your muscles and increase your body's natural ability to move in the full range of motion. When I first began to allow the Core Experience benefit to manifest itself in my life, I found that it allowed me to go further in my flexibility, which automatically increased my range.

You will find out that over a period of time, by using this technique, your overall flexibility will increase.

## 5. Leverage

For any fitness exercise that you do or any type of technique you use, if you find leverage, you've got the advantage.

People ask me, "How do you build lean muscle using dumbbells?" and I tell them that when I am lifting through my core, it provides me with leverage over the weight. Therefore, it is easier for me to take my time and find the positive and negative range. When you find leverage, it is easier to find it through your core. (See figs. 9, 10, and 11 for proper and improper leverage.) That means you're not searching for that leverage. Even when I lift heavy weight, I am confident I can get from A to B if I use my core and this technique to get the balance and the other benefits that come with it. It will help you develop your leverage for any exercise you're looking to do.

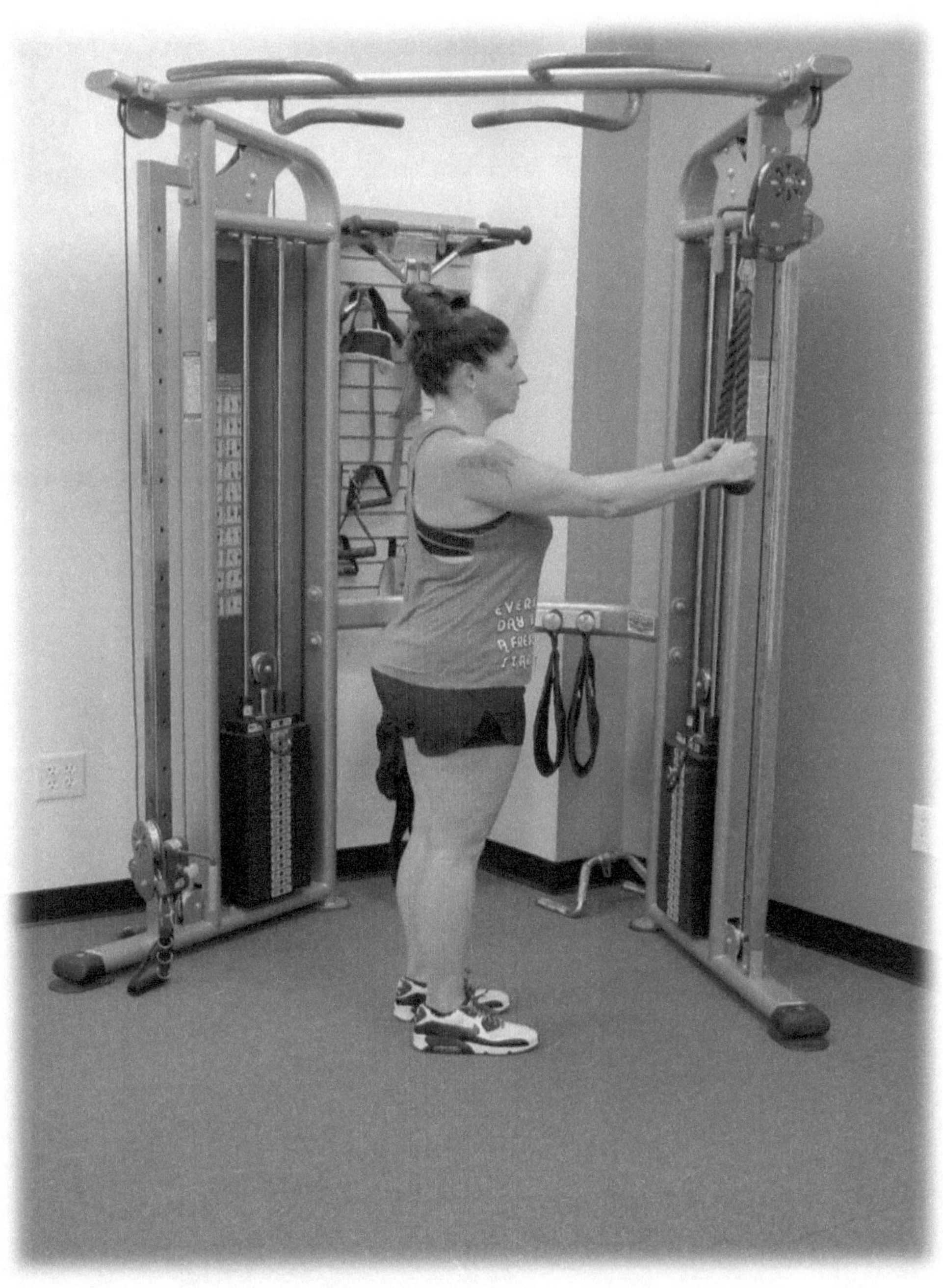

*Figure 9: Improper Triceps Leverage*

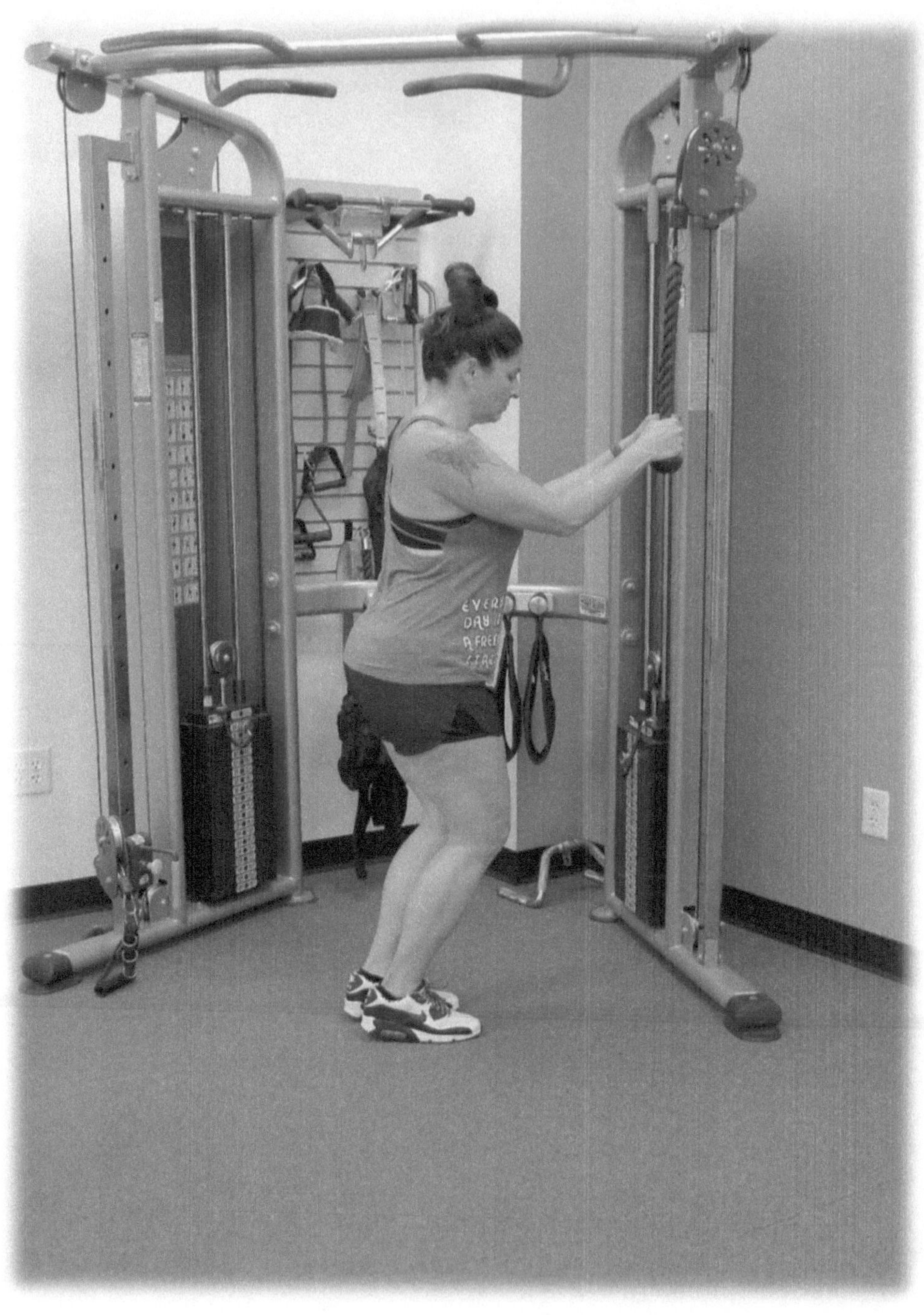

*Figure 10: Proper Core Balance Leverage*

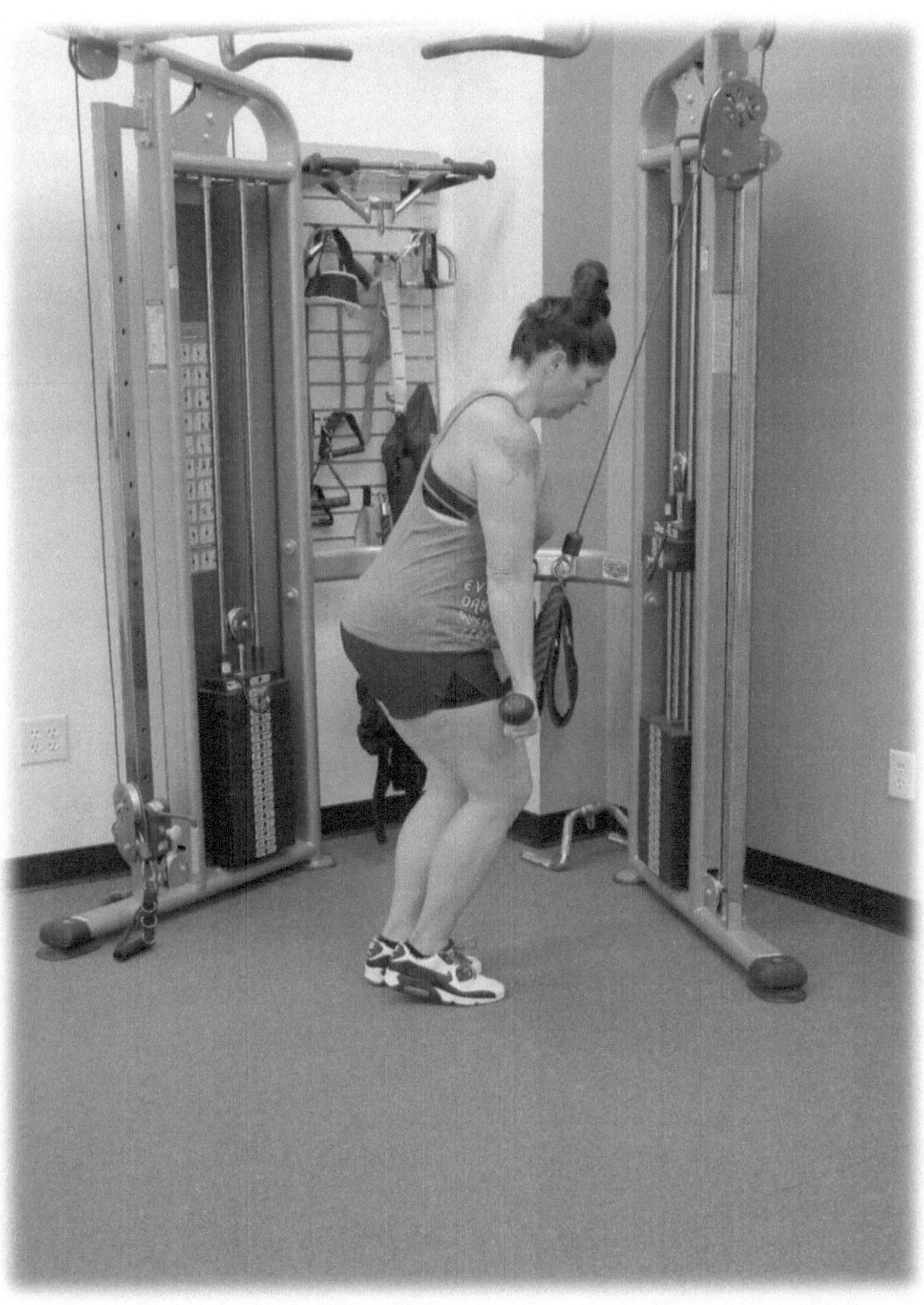

*Figure 11: Proper Core Balance Leverage Triceps Pulldown*

# 6. Balance

Balance is probably the most powerful aspect of the body benefits found in the Core Balance Technique. When you have balance, you have everything.

Balance means that even when you are stationary, your posture is great, and that is exactly what learning the art of this will give you. You'll have balance in every lift you do, whether it's a chest press or something over your shoulders. When you have balance, it means your core really has centered the exercise. This allows you to lift through the power of your core, giving you perfect range from A to B (figs. 13 and 14).

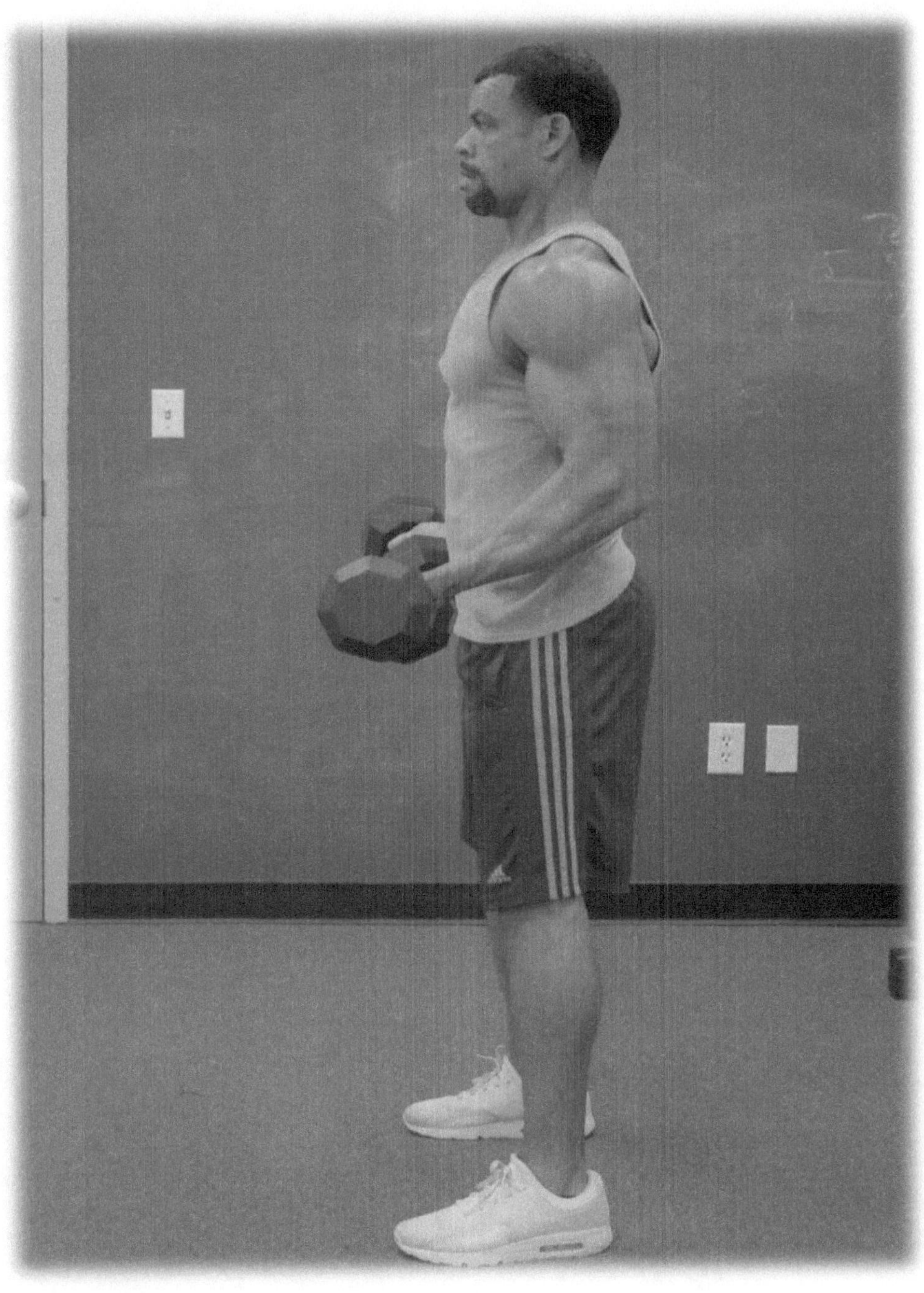

*Figure 12:  Improper Balance*

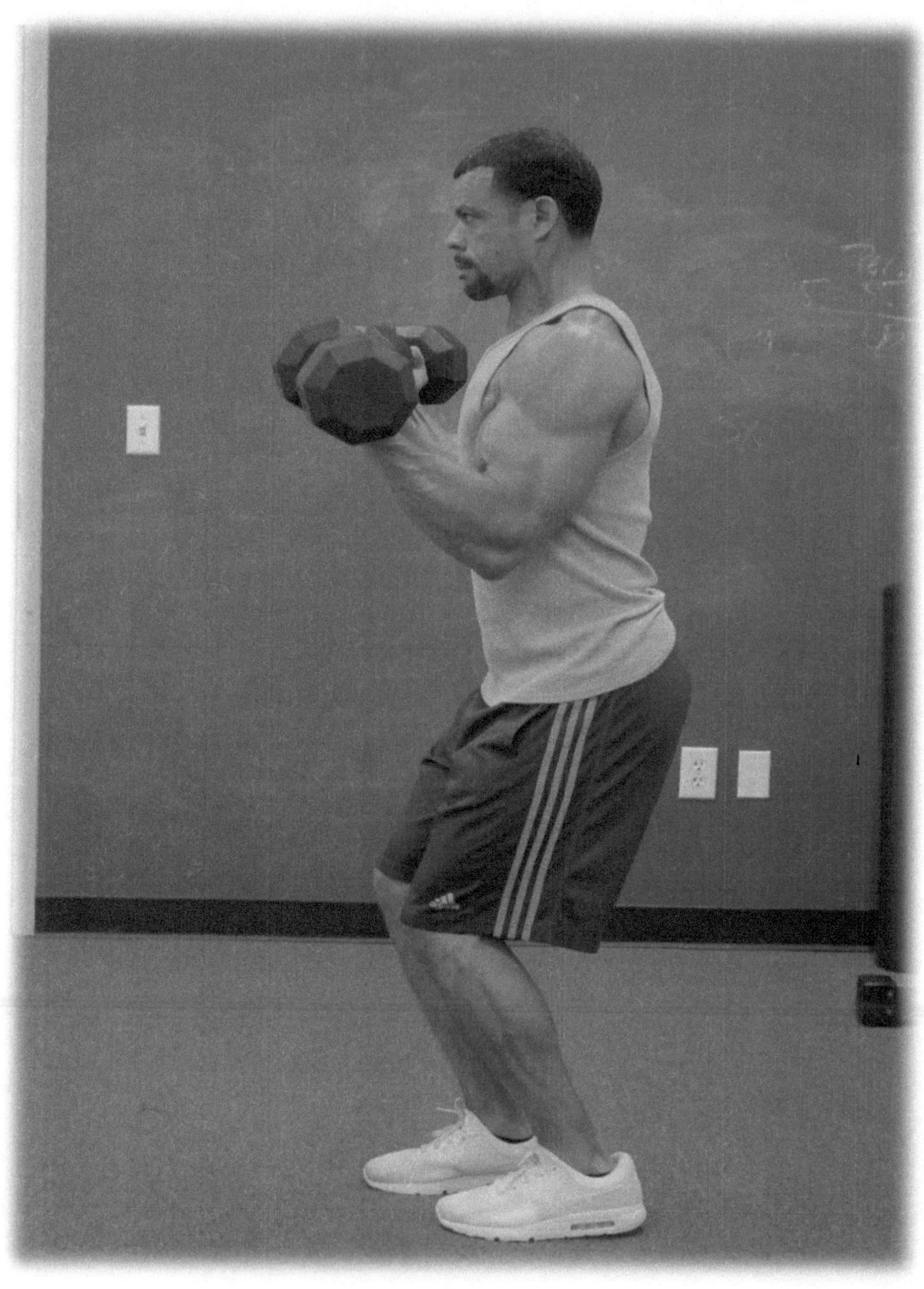

*Figure 13: Proper Core Balance*

Here is why this is important: In my experience, when the balance is not right in my exercise, I have to shift the weight down to get the balance or I will not do the exercise. I simply just do not do any exercise that does not agree with my core and does not allow me to flow in a certain amount of range. However, the advantage is that the actual exercise is not what I'm focusing on. My focus is my technique, regardless of the exercise I do. Once I find the balance of an exercise through my core, I will flow through that exercise like it's nothing.

Here at Nexxt Level Training, we know that the six benefits we have just talked about in this section—posture, strength, building proper lean muscle, flexibility, leverage, and balance—are the keys for meeting your fitness goals. The combination of these gives you a body experience that is perfectly balanced and will benefit you in all areas of your life.

# The Spiritual Benefits of the Core Balance Technique

In this section, we are going to talk about the third benefit of the Core Balance Experience: the spiritual benefit. As we've mentioned before, the Core Balance Technique brings three main benefits to your life: benefits in your body, mind, and spirit.

I am a Christian. I believe in Jesus Christ and completely place my faith and trust in Him. Jesus is my Lord and Savior, which means that as my Lord, He is in control of my life. I follow Him through the leading of the Holy Spirit, whom I believe lives within me. My body is His temple (1 Corinthians 6:19). My relationship with God is a connection that validates my purpose, in the daily walk of my life and also in my fitness journey. This connection provides me with appropriate direction from God, keeping me on the right path. Knowing I am following God's path brings me peace for the journey. God's peace empowers me to set and fulfill my fitness goals on a completely new level, and to understand why I am doing it. I believe that He will do the same for you.

Our goal in taking you through the Core Balance Experience is not only to help you become more physically and mentally strong, but also to build you in spiritual knowledge and strength.

I believe the spiritual aspect of my program is the most important benefit of the three. Let me explain why. Your spirit is the very essence of who you are as a person. It is the process of combining the spiritual aspect of who you are with the goals you have from a fitness standpoint, the physical aspect, and the gains you will make from it to create perfect balance. This is what I like to call a *flow*. In my fitness company, Nexxt Level Training, I am very intentional when working with my clients to focus on the mind, body, and spirit. I clearly believe that the three components must work hand in hand. This flow empowers you to set and reach goals, regardless of the roadblocks you may encounter along the path of the journey.

You have great power within you! Inside of every person, there is passion, a burning desire to thrive and excel. This is connected to your purpose. I do not believe that you "just happened" to wake up one morning wanting to feel better, hoping you could get in shape or to be in good health. There is a spiritual component that fuels your thoughts and feelings. My personal belief is that these are promptings from the Holy Spirit. This is why I suggest that the spiritual aspect of the Core Balance Experience is the most important. The Holy Spirit is the fire burning inside of you, giving you the passion and a sense of urgency to achieve optimal wellness. It empowers you to thrive while accomplishing your goals, and it validates your purpose through the six weeks of the Core Balance Experience.

The following sections break down the spiritual benefits you will see with the Core Balance Experience, and how to combine your goals with your purpose. As a Christian, I believe the Word of God is the basis for understanding all things, including fitness goals. We will begin by laying our foundation on the verse of Romans 8:28 (AMP), which says, "And we know [with great confidence] that God [who is deeply concerned about us] causes all things to work together [as a plan] for good for those who love God, to those who are called according to His plan *and* purpose."

# 1. Connecting Your Goals with God's Purpose

When focusing on how to combine your goals with your purpose, the first step is understanding your purpose through your relationship with God. Because you are in a relationship with God, through Jesus Christ as your Lord and Savior, your spiritual connection will automatically unite your purpose with your goals. Let me tell you the biggest and best part of this. I understand that God is the facilitator of my life, so once my purpose in fitness is connected to His purpose, He gets involved to assist me with completing it. And that's when things really flow to another level. He is, as my Lord, taking control and leading me through the process of fulfilling my purpose and meeting my goals. This is comforting as a believer in Christ. Let me simplify it a little more.

I train many different people. Obviously, each of them have many different goals and things in their lives they desire to accomplish or change. I know that I must address the spiritual needs in their life, so I have to find out where they stand in relationship to God. I personally believe that Jesus Christ is the only way to God the Father. So, if a client already has this foundational belief, we build on that faith knowing we can come into agreement with one another for wisdom, strength, and direction from the Holy Spirit. We can find Bible verses that align with each goal and phase of meeting it. If their belief is not there yet, I must take a different approach. Meeting goals is not a clear path, and it will become difficult throughout the journey. I need to know if they have faith in God on one level or another. I need to know where they will draw their strength from and what will be establishing their thoughts and mindset. I search out if they use Scripture to encourage themselves, or what additional positive methods they utilize in supporting themselves through the tough times.

I always want to find out a person's purpose, plan, and reasoning when setting a greater goal. It is important that we connect the purpose with the journey, as this facilitates the highs and the lows. I will ask specific questions: "What do you want these goals to diversify into?" "How is it going to fit into your current lifestyle?" "How will it affect your family/community?" Having the knowledge of these answers will allow me to find focal points for regrouping through the six-week journey. Regrouping WILL be necessary because when you start fitness training and look at setting and achieving your goals, you will run into some obstacles.

We talked earlier about people *plateauing* in their fitness. By *plateau*, I mean things level out or flatline. They hit a point in the journey where their weight loss may have been three to seven pounds in the first week or two, and now they are stuck at the same weight or losing substantially less over the course of a week. This is very common, and when people plateau, they get frustrated. The frustration will usually produce one of two outcomes: (1) it will ignite a fire that fuels their passion and determination, pushing them harder to excel, or (2) they give up and quit. I often find people right in the middle point. This is the time to remind them of their goals and look at what has already been accomplished. I speak words of encouragement and use this opportunity for spiritual growth.

I can encourage them by sharing the things that I found worked for me personally during my tough times, my lows and struggles, because I too plateaued. I tell them, "When your God-given purpose is connected to your fitness goals, your spirit will push you toward reaching your goals."

I do not care which physical aspect you are challenged with—losing weight, getting stronger, or simply the motivation to work out. I am confident that everything will work out because the spirit is working within you. The benefits of the mind and the body will work in conjunction with your spiritual enlightenment to push you forward in meeting your goals.

I believe this to be true because the Bible says in 1 John 4:4 (NKJV), "He who is in you is greater than he who is in the world." There is a power inside of me that propels me forward in reaching my goals. It is my relationship with Jesus. I take this very seriously because it allows my workouts and everything I do relating to fitness to become a ministry for me. Firstly, it ministers unto me, because my relationship with Christ is a connection that facilitates how I want to open the doors to various workouts and how I am going to push through them in my times of fatigue. On the back end, there is a spiritual enlightenment represented through me, which creates a journey every time I go to the gym. This is not just a workout to me; it is the relationship with God that connects to my purpose.

## 2. Creating a Vision for the Path

The second benefit of the Core Balance Experience is finding a vision for the path of your journey. When I say *vision*, I literally mean being able to imagine or visualize exactly what you hope the fruits produced from your labor will look like. Regardless of what your goal is, if you can visualize yourself at the thirty-day and sixty-day mark, you have vison for your path. Once you have created this image within yourself, you are going to be motivated and committed to pushing yourself continually to the other end. When you have the vison, you will have the needed focal point to direct your fitness goals on the path. Say that you want to lose weight and then visualize being smaller, and watch the created image within yourself successfully walk to the end of the path. This imagery and focus will assist you during your times of frustration and discouragement. Therefore, when you get frustrated during the course of the path, because you can see yourself at that place, with that purpose, meeting that goal, then there is an extra push from within your spirit working to assist you in getting all the way through the process and getting to the end of the path.

Nothing comes without a process. The process will have highs and lows, but when you have vision, you can get through the process. Your vision will enable you to reach your goals, which you are zeroed into at the end of the path. The Bible says, "Where there is no vision, the people perish" (Proverbs 29:18, KJV). That means that where there is no vision, people quit. People will give up and quit right in the middle of the process. I cannot count how many times I have found myself struggling to get where I wanted to go, either in my fitness goals or in an area of trying to achieve a life principle, because I lacked the vision of the end result. Every successful plan requires a vision.

When you have faith in God, when you have faith in Jesus and faith in the power of the Holy Spirit, then the Bible will give you the vision. The Spirit of God will provide you with the vison of what it will look like to reach that goal. Not only will He give you the vision of that goal, but He will also help you with it! This is the power of being able to walk by faith with God when it comes down to fitness. God desires for you to be in the best shape, to be structurally strong. God desires for you to be empowered in your mind, body, and spirit. When you build a relationship with Him, when you are depending on His Spirit,

He will walk you down that path. Whether that be in righteousness or in "the valley of the shadow of death" the Bible says, "[You] will fear no evil" (Psalms 23:4, KJV). Through Christ Jesus, there is no challenge within your body that cannot be accomplished; not in weight loss, not in mental clarity or any physical ailments. The path has already been written with the spiritual enlightenment for you based on your relationship with God.

## 3. Peace

Third, you will benefit from peace with the Core Balance Experience. When you place your faith and dependence on God, you are completely trusting in the Lord. You are not relying on your ability to make things happen; it is 100 percent the power of the Holy Spirit. This ensures you can walk down this path being confident you are supplied with what it takes to get your goals accomplished. Isaiah 26:3 (ESV) states, "You keep him in perfect peace whose mind is stayed on you, because he trusts in you." When you believe this passage of Scripture, you can set a thirty-day or sixty-day goal with peace on your mind.

The peace of God allots your purpose and vision to follow the flow of the Holy Spirit. You can see a mountain in front of you and not be detoured. It will not matter what obstacle attempts to block your vision; you will remain focused and at peace. I am confident in this because the Word says so in Philippians 4:6 (NIV): "And the peace of God, which transcends all understanding, will guard your hearts and your minds in Christ Jesus." Your relationship with Jesus is your connection between the beginning and the end of your journey. He is the Alpha and the Omega, the beginning and the end (Revelation 1:18). When you have spiritual enlightenment and you believe in the Word of God, it will allow you to understand that the end has already been established. The end result and successes of your fitness journey were established before you even thought about beginning, through Christ Jesus. That is a great revelation to have. Now you may ask yourself, how does this fit into Core Balance?

Core Balance does everything from the center. It gives you balance and proportion, and your faith will help you maintain balance because of your relationship with God. When you get the balance of peace, you will automatically get what the Bible calls *rest*. When you have that peace and that rest working in your life, God will help you get through every stage. He will help transform your mind, He will help transform your body, and He will help transform your spirit through perfect peace to a place where you walk to the goals you have set.

## 4. Fulfillment

Spiritual fulfillment is like a second wind inside of a workout. When you understand that there's a shift because of your efforts, you will get fulfillment. You can see the light at the end of the tunnel, even in the crazy mix of the process of where you are working so hard to get. I can tell you that when you get spiritual fulfillment, nothing is going to turn you back. Nothing will prevent you from reaching that goal.

Because you have a relationship with God, you know that there's a power greater than your humanity and own abilities to accomplish things. You understand that the power of the Holy Spirit is also pushing you to get through to your goal. Your body and mind will follow in line to the subjection of what spirituality is driving: the burning and passionate desire to attain your fitness goals.

At Nexxt Level Training, we build our whole principle and faith on the purpose of God. We believe that if we intend on building one part of a human being, it is necessary to build all parts—their minds, bodies and spirits. This is the reason we teach Core Balance: we teach the benefits for achieving total wellness. This fulfillment aspect will give you the stage to walk to the very end of what you see at the beginning. With that said, the spiritual benefit of being in a relationship with God will provide you with the wisdom needed to make sense of everything you are looking for.

The Bible says, "Wisdom is the principal thing; therefore get wisdom: and with all your getting get understanding" (Proverbs 4:7, KJV). When you understand that it is God's passion and heart for you to be healthy, to be in the best shape of your life, and to be structurally strong, you can walk out your vision and purpose in peace. That means inside of you, you can feel good about the purpose God has for you. You can walk with confidence, understanding that spiritually you have been empowered and should feel good about yourself. Your identity, all by itself because it is in Christ, will push you to the next level in fitness and in your daily life.

Now that you have learned about the third benefit of the Core Balance Experience, being built spiritually, it's time to move on and talk about the Core Balance System itself.

# The Core Balance System

This section will be about the Core Balance *System*. With every program or idea, there has to be a system. This system is how you get from A to Z. With every client, I draw a path for them to get to their goals. With my twenty years of experience, I have learned how to use this system for different workouts and build proportional lean muscle. This system has provided me with everything I need, and I can tweak it in many different ways. I will talk you through this system and the workouts in it, so you can get the results you want.

The system consist of six major workouts:

## 1. The Measuring Stick

In this workout, you do a circuit where the same number of reps is done for each exercise in the circuit. For example, if one of my clients can do ten repetitions of an exercise, I will make ten reps the standard across the board, for every exercise they do. By setting this number, I can measure where the client's strength is at ten repetitions, as well as measure their technique. This is a good starting point when beginning the Core Balance Experience, and ten repetitions of each exercise is very convenient because it's not too much or too little.

When you are using this technique, it is easy to find out what a set of ten looks like. The measuring stick will give you a smooth transition to our next workout: the downstairs walk.

## 2. The Downstairs Walk

The next workout is called the downstairs walk because with every set, you will decrease the number of repetitions. For example, if you start with twelve repetitions, the next step will be ten, the next will be eight, and so on. The resistance will be increased as you go down in reps, and I will check to see where your technique is as you walk down those steps.

This allows me to see where your base is and how the Core Balance Technique will hold as you increase the resistance you put on. This is powerful because you can shake this up in many different ways. It does not have to be twelve, ten, and eight reps; it could also be twelve, ten, five, and five.

The important thing is where your energy is and what level of technique you are able to hold as you put more resistance on. The more resistance you put on, the higher your heart rate and the more calories you will burn.

It will teach you how to be efficient when your heart rate is up and stay within the confines of what you're doing in your workout. It will help you get stronger, test the foundations of your technique, and burn more calories.

### 3. **Crazy 8s**

In the third week of workouts, each set will consist of eight reps.

This number is below ten and above six. Doing just eight reps allows me to put a little more resistance into the workouts. It is called *crazy 8s* because as you go from one set to the other set it will get harder and harder, because additionally, your rest period will be cut in half.

What is beautiful about this is that as long as I do eight repetitions, I do not care about the weight. As long as your technique is clean and the intervals of rest are shorter between the reps, it will help you burn more calories, get stronger, and begin to shred excess pounds and fat as you are training.

## 4. **Drop-Off Set**

This is the workout that will determine where your commitment really is as far as your goals. This exercise will challenge everything you have learned in the last three weeks and will be the one that will solidify this work. It brings in cardio and high heart rate and gives you strength at the same time.

To do a drop-off set you are going to do the following:

Start with twelve repetitions and then take the weight down and in the same set do ten repetitions. Then take the weight down again and do five repetitions. To finish, the fourth set is a combination of using minimal weight with fifteen repetitions. That's a lot of repetitions in one set. This will test every bit of strength, endurance, and everything you have gathered in the first three weeks of work.

Additionally, it will also solidify your strength because it will show you where your technique starts and where it begins to break down. The main purpose for this particular workout is to build and test your endurance. You will literally be doing twenty to thirty reps of one exercise, so it requires some mental preparation. Your mentality will enable your body to find something extra that you did not know you had! Once you get into the second or third set, you will find a second wind that boosts your ability to push through to the final sets.

## 5. Long-Distance Run

In this workout you will take all the weight down and bring the repetitions up. Ultimately, you will be doing three sets of twenty to twenty-five reps per muscle while transitioning through various exercises. For example, if you are doing the arms, you would do twenty to twenty-five bicep curls, then do twenty to twenty-five triceps pulldowns, and then twenty to twenty-five dips.

You want to do a high number of repetitions for each exercise in your workout. That will keep you in the middle of what you did last week with the drop-out sets and what you will do next week, where we increase the weights. The long-distance run is a workout that tests your endurance. You're not doing that much weight, but you are doing almost double the repetitions. Once you get up into those areas of twenty to twenty-five reps, you will really start finding those fatigue areas.

## 6. The Weight Workout

Here is where you really test the foundation of the resistance you have built over the entire program.

Here's how you do it: You will usually do twelve, eight, five, and five repetitions. Every time you do twelve, test out how much weight you can handle comfortably. Then, drop to eight repetitions and go up in weight. When you get to five and five, take your weight up almost as much as you can handle. Here, your technique will still help you bear the weight you are holding.

I tell my clients that a house is usually as strong as its foundation. So if you put too much weight on the foundation, it will crack and shake.

Week five prepares you for what you are doing in this week, week six. This workout is to test the resistance you have built throughout the other five weeks. It is fun and gratifying because at this point you can compare where you were at the beginning and where you are now.

Once you are done with week six, you will understand the journey it took to go through every single one of those workouts, and you will gain confidence as well as improve your mindset going forward. You will know how much your foundation will hold, and you can begin to build on top of that.

As you can now see, the Core Balance Experience is a six-week workout system where each week builds on top of the previous week. It does not matter whether you train two, three, four, or five times a week, this system will work for you. The six-week program is realistic and easy to wrap your mind around verses something longer. This allows you to learn the technique from week one to week six and get great value at the end of the six weeks. This is the Core Balance System.

# The Fruits of the Core Balance Experience

In this section, I want to go over the fruits of the Core Balance Experience. These are very important to anybody who wants to take this technique, begins to use it, and learn the heart of it. The truth is, there are so many different ways Core Balance is going to help you, whether you do your workouts in the gym or at home. Not only that, but as we have discussed before, you will be able to bring these benefits into your personal life as well. The following are just some of the fruits you will enjoy from the work you put into this system:

1. **Your workout should become cleaner.**

Once you begin to focus on your core and the core begins to dominate the range of the different exercises you do—no matter the circuit—your workouts will become cleaner. What this means is that you will not feel obligated to build resistance here or there. Instead, you will have a clean range of workouts with these exercises EVEN if your heart is at an accelerated rate.

Once your workouts become cleaner, it creates what I call a *flow*. When you are able to flow from exercise to exercise, your workouts become cleaner. You are not fighting different exercises to try to go from one point to another. When you start an exercise, you can use your technique, so then you can flow from A to B to C.

## 2. Your workouts should become shorter.

Once your workouts become cleaner and once you understand that you bring more value to the equipment than the equipment brings to you, you will give the workout more value than what it gives you. The stability of Core Balance will begin to dominate these workouts. Then you won't have to work out in the gym all day to get results. I'm not a big believer in going to the gym for two hours every day. That is just not realistic for most people. My workouts are five days a week, forty to fifty minutes max. So in about fifty minutes I know I'll be leaving the gym.

One of the big plusses for me has been that because I've been able to learn and master this technique, I know what my body wants. As you begin to implement this technique, you begin to know when you need to taper things off and when you need to stop your workout. It's not easy to explain this feeling, but when I use the Core Balance Technique my workouts become cleaner and much shorter.

## 3. It helps you be efficient when your heart rate is at an accelerated pace.

What I have learned with Core Balance is that when I dominate everything with my core, I can quickly move from exercise to exercise. There is something in the fitness industry that we call *super set*. A *super set* is when you do one exercise and combine it with another and another. The Core Balance Technique allows you to dominate the *super set*. You can do an exercise, get your heart rate up to burn calories, and not have to stop and take elongated rests, keeping your heart at an accelerated rate. I think taking long breaks between sets is a detriment to a workout.

The flow that is created while using this technique allows you to go from workout to workout, even as you feel your heart rate up. This way you're still able to shift and be efficient. What this does is combine cardio and efficiency while your heart rate is up, thus burning more calories. You are also still giving it a certain amount of resistance with the various exercises. All of this working together is an awesome experience.

## 4. The Core Balance Technique helps you maximize space.

Sometimes when you do workouts, you're all over the gym. However, when you learn how to use Core Balance, you can use a small space, bring a certain amount of equipment into that space, and maximize it. There are so many exercises you can do with the Core Balance Technique that you can do in a small space, using a few weights or dumbbells to increase the intensity of the exercise. This is awesome for those that go to gyms that are very populated and busy, because now you can take a certain space and make the most of it. With the limited amount of space and just a few tools, you will accomplish the same results you could going from machine to machine. That also makes your workouts cleaner and much shorter.

These fruits are powerful because once you learn how to make things cleaner, it will carry over to your lifestyle and how you manage things. For example, you will learn how to maximize other things, like your time.

This leads me back to point number two. The same way you can get into a gym and work out clean and short, you can also maximize time in your business. If you know you don't have to be in the gym all day, you will be able to fit more into your schedule. If you are like most people, you are busy, and once you can fit fitness into your schedule, you become more efficient.

Being efficient and being able to be efficient with an accelerated heart rate lets you know that when things get chaotic and busy you can still be efficient. This keeps you from quitting. It gives you a mindset where you understand that even though all of these thing are happening, all you have to do is really handle them just like you handle things when training.

In your everyday life, you have to maximize spaces of time, areas, and many more things. It doesn't take much time to fit in the things that are necessary.

When we talk about the fruits of the Core Balance Technique, we are talking about a benefit that is going to take you a long way. I want you to be efficient in a weight room, not just efficient in training at home. I want you to be able to pull these principles from the Core Balance Experience and use them in your life. It will make you a better person, it will make you commit to your purposes, and make things work better for what you are trying to accomplish.

# Thank You

In closing, I want to express my heartfelt gratitude for your decision to purchase my book. Not only do I want to thank you for spending your financial resources and time reading *The Core Balance Experience*, but also for allowing me to communicate my personal journey through the process of writing it. Again, I truly believe the Core Balance Experience is more than a fitness experience; it is a life experience.

The art of this technique, the principles I have built it on, and its versatility are life changing. My goal in sharing the Core Balance Experience with others is to help people obtain total health and fitness. Optimal health requires more than simply being physically fit. Wholeness comes when the mind, body, and spirit are all three working in unity and balance. The basis for my content throughout this book is found in my faith in Jesus

Christ and His Word. The Bible says that when your mind is focused on the Lord, you will have perfect peace (Isaiah 26:3). He will give you the ability to do all things (Philippians 4:13), and He will restore your health (Jeremiah 30:17). I pray this will be a transitioning place in your life and that these materials will help take you to The Nexxt Level. Find more information and resources on my website @ www.nexxtleveltraining.com.